PART ONE

CHAPTER

1

This book is dedicated to my mother Karen.

Copyright Notice/Legal Disclaimer

How You Can Save Big Money On Medical Expenses!

By Brian Orvik

Copyright Brian Orvik 2019

This book is a reference guide, not a medical guide. It is not a guide for medical self-diagnosis or self treatment. You should always consult a doctor about your medical matters. This book should not be used as a substitute for medical consultation.

This book is designed to help people lower the costs of their medical expenses. I do not and will not benefit financially by mentioning or endorsing any company, institution or product in this book (other than my own books).

The consumer needs to investigate any and all information concerning their medical needs. Any information given in this book about companies or institutions I suggest, needs to be investigated by the consumer. The author has no liability or responsibility for decisions made by people who read anything printed in this book. Facts and information and websites may change. Laws, policies and procedures of medical insurances and policies may change. Please use due diligence in your medical research.

I'm not a doctor or lawyer. Consult you lawyer about any legal or tax matters. Consult your doctor about any medical matters. Before beginning any exercise program you should consult your doctor. Before taking any supplements you should consult your doctor and pharmacist, especially if you are already taking medications.

2

Table Of Contents

How You Can Save Big Money On Medical Expenses!

Orvik…pg 103

3

Medical Shopping And Prevention Are The Best Medicines

America has a serious problem. It is our huge deficit brought about, in part, by the expenses of Medicare and Medicaid. These 2 programs accounted for approximately 26% of federal spending in 2018. It should be growing to an even larger percentage as more baby boomer's retire. This is a serious problem that our Congress refuses to address. You and I will have to be the ones that get sanity back into the medical marketplace by making wise choices to steer

our health care industry down its true
correct path.

If people would use the suggestions that
are in this book, then eventually medical
care costs would go down. If Medicaid and
insurance companies didn't, for example,
pay $5,000 for hearing aids, then the prices
for them would go down. If you and I
wouldn't spend $5,000 for hearing aids, then
why would our government? Even if you
have an insurance program that will pay
$5,000 for hearing aids, it is in your, mine
and our best interest to find the cheapest
hearing aids (that work well for us) for 2
reasons.

The first reason is that if the costs go down
for each person's medical expenditures, then
the cost of the total insurance
premiums/costs will eventually go down for
everyone. This is true for private and public
insurance programs. This in the end, would
save you money on your taxes and/or your
health insurance premiums/costs. If you
don't have insurance, then the total savings
would go directly into your pocket.

The second reason for searching around to get the lowest cost of your health care goods and services is that if every one went and got a colonoscopy for $1,100 (for example), eventually the crooks who charge $9,000 would have to lower their prices or go out of business. We need to get ourselves back into the circle of medical price decision makers. Then the LAW of supply and demand will start working in the health care industry again.

One of the things that makes America great is the free enterprise system. It is mostly based on supply and demand. Therefore, in our society the prices of goods and services generally will go to its natural, normal and fair level (and the quality also usually goes up). When the government "helps" with programs, that's when we generally have problems. Medicare, for the most part, sets the prices of medical procedures and costs in America. When a third party, whether it is government or insurance companies, pays for the end results then the natural free market tendency to "shop around" for prices goes out the window. When the the government says "we'll pay $5,000 for hearing aids", they are setting the prices for our health care, not the free market or us. Now there are also other reasons costs are high for health care in America.

Insurance, regulations/paperwork and administrative personnel also add costs to our medical expenses. These costs are hard to avoid unless you go to a clinic or hospital that don't use government and/or private insurance. I'll be talking about 2 cost reducing medical providers, Direct Primary Care and Micro Hospitals, in later chapters.

People think insurance companies rip them off. Obviously they are in business to make money. But it is mostly pharmaceutical companies and hospitals that charge astronomical prices for goods and services. Government and insurance companies just enable them. Health insurance spreads the risk of health care costs over a group of people. Insurance companies are regulated by each state, and like casinos, they are only allowed to make a certain percentage of profit on their total sales. So they aren't directly charging you outrageous prices.

They gouge you indirectly because they have little incentive to keep costs down since a 8% profit on $1 billion is better than a 8% profit on $1 million. This aspect of insurance needs addressing.

America spends way more money than any other country on it's medical costs. Not until we get government and insurance companies mostly out of medicine, will prices for medical expenses go back to where supply and demand dictate that they should naturally be at. Only by having the consumer shopping around for their own medical goods and services (like most everything else they purchase) will the cost of our medical care and expenses go down.

We will discuss ways that you can save on your health care costs throughout this book. In this chapter I'd like to also focus on another thing that would greatly reduce the costs of medical care for everyone in the U.S., prevention. About 67% of the adult population in the U.S. is overweight, about 39% of the adult population is obese. This in turn creates all kinds of medical problems for our citizens. High blood pressure, type 2 diabetes, high cholesterol (heart disease) and other chronic illnesses raise the costs of medicine unbelievably and unnecessarily high.

Estimates are that about 1/3 of Americans have high blood pressure. The costs of high blood pressure in America are reported to be anywhere from $100-$200 billion a year. The costs of diabetes are estimated to be from $100-$250 billion a year. Whether you as the tax payer pay for these costs or you as an employee pay for these costs in lesser wages and/or higher copays and deductibles, it doesn't matter.

If everyone in this country were to get to their correct weight, and stay there, our medical expenses would drastically drop. Not only would people feel and look better, but the costs spent on Medicaid, Medicare and private health insurance would drop greatly. This would lead you and I to be paying less in taxes and for our private insurance.

Another way to reduce the costs of health care is by having a yearly physical. This will help find potential health problems before they get out of control. Also, doing your preventive tests such as a colonoscopy or mammogram will also greatly reduce the costs of medical care (and the risk to your life). Prevention and proactive preventive medical care can save tons of cash to the patient and health care consumers in general.

A famous doctor presently on TV recommends taking a daily multi-vitamin, fish oil and calcium/magnesium supplements. These are some of the things that I take daily. You might want to ask your doctor if there are supplements or vitamins that they suggest you take regularly. These might possibly be the simplest and easiest ways to help stay healthy, especially if you don't eat properly.

I was over weight by about 50 lbs. I wrote a book on how I lost the weight. I've been pretty good about keeping my weight off. I no longer have high blood pressure and my diabetes is in remission. My book is called "How I Lost 46 Lbs. In 96 Days" by Brian Orvik. Yes this is a plug, but if I can lose the weight so can you (if you are over weight.) In the book I describe my weight loss journey and the supplements I took to get my conditions under control. The book explains how I used hawthorn berry supplements to help control high blood pressure and cinnamon supplements to help control my type 2 diabetes.

If we'd lose the weight, we'd probably need less medication and medical treatments. So the moral of this chapter is prevention and medical shopping are the best medicines to help save on our outrageously expensive health care costs.

The 2 best ways for us to get the costs of medical expenses down is for us to first get to our correct weight and other prevention activities. Prevention is the number one way. The second way is to shop around. You will probably save directly out of pocket by doing this and we'll start using supply and demand to lower our overall and actual costs of medical goods and services. These are the 2 reasons I wrote this book.

At the beginning of each chapter I'll

discuss ways that you might be able to prevent medical problems in that area of medical concern, before they become a problem. Each chapter is also designed to give you ideas on how you can save money in those different areas of medical expenses.

4

How You Can Save On Dental Expenses

It seems that regardless of whether you have employee dental coverage or if you get coverage from a private insurance company, it will probably cost you about the same price. Some companies pay for their employees dental insurance, but most just allow employees to purchase coverage though their company with deductions from their paycheck. Just turn on your TV and someone will probably try to sell you dental insurance.

It is hard to get cheap dental work or dental insurance in the U.S. But there are a few ways which may work for you to help lower your dental costs. Once again, prevention is the best medicine. Floss every night and then brush your teeth after you floss. Brush after you eat breakfast. Brush for 2 minutes. If you make a habit of doing these things, your dental expenses should be pretty low regardless of how you get your dental care. Think about putting a note on your bathroom mirror to remind you and your family to brush and floss. Reward your kids for brushing and flossing. You just need to get into the habit of doing these preventive dental hygiene acts. If you drink sugary drinks or sodas or eat sugary foods, you should rinse after drinking or eating them (if you can't brush). Sugar is bad for your teeth.

The good thing about employer dental insurance is that it is usually deducted from your check every month, so it is good insurance against huge dental expenses. If you have any insurance whether dental or medical, you should consider using a Flexible Savings Account or Health Savings

Account or Health Reimbursement Account. These programs allow pre-tax dollars to be used for your medical treatments or employer reimbursement. Consult your tax attorney, CPA or human resources personnel about these programs.

Plaque builds up on your teeth and it is bad. You should have it removed twice a year. When I don't have dental insurance I go to the local dental school and they clean my teeth for $40. They can also do x-rays, but since they don't do actual dental work this isn't necessary in my opinion. When you go to the regular dentist they will usually want you to have their x-rays taken anyways.

If you don't have dental insurance you'll probably save money by going to a dental school, since at the dentist's office it should cost you between $150-$250 to get your teeth cleaned. In my state, it is also required to have x-ray's done (or so the dental office tells me) when you go to the dentist. So going to the regular dentist would also require me to get x-ray's, and this would also cost me extra. I get away with little actual dental care because I brush and floss daily. If you don't brush and floss regularly, you probably will be having trouble with your teeth and gums.

Another good thing about going to the dental school is that they usually take their time and your teeth look great afterwords. You're also helping out a future dental hygienist get practice. You can find local dental schools at the web address ada.org/267.aspx. Search for the state that you want and then look for local cities. Then look up hygienist schools. Call up a local dental school and check their prices, then make an appointment.

You can also get actual dental work done at dental schools. You can go to ada.org/267.aspx again and then look for your state and then nearby city. Then look for PREDOC schools or other schools by procedure (periodontics, orthodontics, etc.). Call them up. They are also looking for mouths to work on. I have never did this, but I don't have an actual dentist school near me. I just have a dental hygienist training school in my area that I frequent.

Once when I had dental insurance, I went and had my teeth cleaned by the dental school anyway. My insurance company reimbursed me 80% of the $40. So I got $32 back and it cost me just $8 for the cleaning. This was cheaper than the co-pay at the dentist. Going to a dental school for just cleanings and still having your dental insurance for emergencies, would be a great way to save with cheaper and better cleanings and less x-rays (in my opinion).

Another way I could save on my dental bill is by doing a fluoridation rinse, just like I do at the dental office. The last time I went to the dentist they wanted me to have a fluoride rinse. My insurance company didn't pay for it so it would have cost me $50. If this is the same fluoride I can buy at the store then I could just give myself fluoride treatments as directed on the bottle, and save big money. By the way, my dental school gives me the fluoride rinse included with the $40.

If you do or don't have dental insurance you can look up the costs of local dental procedures at fairhealthconsumer.org or healthcarebluebook.com to get an idea of the costs of dental procedures in your area. When you see a dentist and you are told that you need a certain procedure, before you commit, look up the cost and then negotiate with your dentist to get a better price. Even if you have insurance you should be doing this anyway since it will probably save you money on your deductible or any other costs your insurance might not pay for (like the fluoride treatment).

Also, ask the dentist if the procedure is direly important. It seems like every time I go to the dentist they say "I think we should fill that tooth". I usually just go to the actual dentist about every 5 years. If you really needed a filling I think they'd say "we have to get that filled right away". So ask if it is really necessary. If you have a list of dental procedures the dentist really thinks you need done and you don't have much money, then prioritize what should be done first or ask if you can make payments.

If you are short of cash and don't have or want to use credit cards, there are dentists that take payments. I know two ladies that make payments to their dentist. Ask your current dentist if they'll take payments, if you've been a customer for a long time, they'll probably be receptive. Otherwise, call around to local dental offices and ask if they take payments or search the internet for "dentists near me that take payments". This is for people with or without insurance.

Another way I hear you can save big money on dental costs is by going down to Mexico to get major procedures done. I've never done this, but I know people who have. I'd consider it if I lived close to the border and my American dentist wanted to charge me outrageous prices, which they usually do. Chapter 16 has more information on medical tourism.

You may qualify for free or discounted dental work through NeedyMeds, a non-profit organization. Go to their website and see if you qualify.

There are other programs that also offer free or low cost dental help. Check and see if these websites might be able to help you: freedentalcare.us, freedental.org,

dentallifeline.org or
findahealthcenter.hrsa.gov. You may have to
qualify for some of these programs.

You can find dental insurance through a
site called dentalplans.com. This site might
help you find dental insurance for a cost that
you can afford.

If you are low income, you can contact
your county medical department to see if
you can get free or low cost dental care
through them. In my county we have the
Red River Vally Dental Access Project that is
a county access program for people without
insurance and that have dental pain. I took
this lady I know down there once, it only
cost her $30 and they fixed her up. Try
searching the internet for "social services"
and your county and/or your city and state.
You might also try an internet search for
"free dental" or "low cost dental" and then
enter your county or city and state. There
may be low income requirements to be
eligible for these types of programs.

You may be eligible for free or
discounted dental care through the Veteran's

Administration if you qualify for VA benefits. Go on-line to va.gov or contact your local VA to see if you are eligible. If you are eligible for Medicaid, you might also get dental coverage for free or discounted care. You can see if you are eligible for Medicaid by going to your state's Medicaid eligibility website. Search by your state and "Medicaid" on the internet. I'm not aware of Medicare offering dental plans. Apparently 65% of the elderly don't have any form of dental insurance.

Always consult your dentist about any dental problems and preventive care.

5

How You Can Save On Chiropractors

The best way to save on back and neck pain costs is prevention. If you have to move a heavy or bulky item, get help. Use your knees when you pick things up, not your back. Keep the thing your moving next to you, don't hold it far away from your body. Do not twist when you are carrying something heavy. Don't jump off of high places and land. I think running has done damage to my back and knees. If you workout, try to do exercises that don't require continual jolting to your back and knees. Being at your correct weight will take a lot of strain off your back and knees. Try to have good posture, don't hunch over. By doing these things, hopefully you won't have problems with your back, neck, knees and body.

When I was a kid my uncle told me that he had 4 back surgeries. He told me, "don't ever have back surgery". I've tried to remember his advice over the years.

Back and neck problems can give you great discomfort. If you've ever had back or neck pain, you know what I'm talking about. When I was younger I was in the Army and jumped out of planes. The training and actual jumping caused constant jarring to my back and knees, this led to years of pain. The many years I've spent running 1000's of miles probably hasn't helped my back and knees either. I've only been to the chiropractor once. My knee was acting up and I thought he could help me. But he said it was arthritis and he couldn't do anything for me.

Since then I've had x-rays of my back and

knees and they have confirmed that I do have arthritis in them. I thought my back pains might have had much more serious problems. The x-rays didn't show this though. I first began having back and neck pain not too long after getting out of the military. When I was leaving the Army the military separation guy told me that since I was a paratrooper that my back was messed up, I just didn't know it yet. I thought he was crazy. Within 2 years I was in pain. I didn't want to go to the VA or go to a chiropractor though.

I decided to read books on how to get my back better. They usually prescribed doing exercises to strengthen my back muscles. I wasn't going to do this since I was being lazy. So I just hoped that my back wouldn't give me pain and trouble.

I thought to myself, if I could hang upside down then it would probably pop my back and neck back into place. Did I mention that I'd been in horrible horrendous pain and wasn't even able to turn my head sometimes. I went down to a shop and looked at some inversion tables to hang upside down with, but back then they wanted about $1500 for them. I guess I didn't need help that bad. Then I bought my first house and put a pull up bar in the back yard. I bought a pair of inversion boots for $40 and preceded to hang up side down on the bar whenever my back was out of alignment. This solved my problem, until the next time I needed to hang upside down. Later I bought an inversion table at a yard sale. This was a prescription one (top notch) for only $75.

Recently I bought a second, new inversion table on-line for $120. It took me a couple of hours to put together, but it is great. Whenever my back and/or neck give me problems, I just hang upside down. Not for too long because the blood rushes to my head. This usually does the trick for me.

I'd advise anyone to try an inversion table if they are having back or neck problems. You should talk to your doctor first, especially if you are over weight or have had knee, back or neck surgery. But hanging upside down has worked for me for over 25 years.

I didn't have access to my inversion table for a while years ago and my back started acting up. I did have a gym membership though so I thought I'd try find relief down at the club. I went over to the weight's area and got on a pulley weight machine and set the weights at heavy. I pulled down on the bar. Then I let the weights pull my spine up. This makes it a sort of an inverted inversion machine. It pulled my spine up and I got relief from that. So if you belong to a gym I suggest you also try that out if you're having back problems, after talking to your doctor.

In the past when I've had problems with my back and neck I've found that swimming often times helps put my back into place. You also could try this if you have back and neck problems.

Years ago I hurt the arch of my left foot. Sometimes I still have horrendous pain there, especially when I wear the wrong shoes. When you are limping, it throws your whole body out of whack/alignment. I went down to one of the nation's largest foot stores that make plastic arch supports. I spent good money for these custom hard plastic arch supports 15 years ago. But it has saved me from horrible pain over the years. I still have them and use them when my arches give me trouble. If you have feet or arch issues, seriously consider getting these custom made plastic arch shoe supports. I told someone how much the arch supports cost and they said "that's too much". If you are in horrible pain, how much would you pay for it to go away? Back then I think I paid about $250 for the pair of arch supports.

If you live close to an accredited chiropractic college, you might get cheap treatments through them. Search the internet for "chiropractic schools" or "chiropractic colleges" and then your city/state.

Chiropractors tend to be not as expensive as doctors and dentists, so having insurance might not be as necessary to have for them. Care from them shouldn't be out of reach for most people if needed. Most chiropractors take insurance though. If you have medical insurance, make sure the chiropractor you wish to go to is a network provider for your insurance company. You should check to see if your insurance covers chiropractors, how much of a co-pay you'll have and how many times they'll cover you to go to see one in a year. You don't need a surprise medical bill.

If you are having back, neck, feet or knee problems, consult your doctor.

6

How You Can Save On Vision Care

Many times your vision insurance is free or costs you a monthly deduction through your employer. You can also get private insurance from TV ads or insurance companies. There are mostly 3 types of problems with vision. Nearsightedness and/or farsightedness. If you are farsighted, this is good. If you are nearsighted you'll probably need to see an eye doctor.

I want to mention here that your vision troubles could be some other problem, perhaps serious. It could be   a sign of diabetes, glaucoma or something else. It would be best for you to determine what the real cause of your vision problems are first, before you get glasses. You should see a doctor or an eye doctor before you just buy glasses. But for me, my need for glasses was just old eyes.

As far as prevention goes, when I was a kid my parents used to say "don't watch TV with the lights out". I thought that was sort of stupid. But I mostly complied, when they were around. Later I read a medical article on this subject. Yes, scientifically, you shouldn't watch TV with the lights off. The science of it is hard to explain, so I'm not going to try explain it. Also, if you're reading, use a bright light bulb, don't strain your eyes. When you are on-line have the lights on in the room and have the computer screen bright.

It seemed like the day I turned 40, my vision started to go. I can still see far away (so I'm farsighted), but I can't read small letters very well. Every year it gets worse. Instead of going to the eye doctor repeatedly

I've just bought my corrective lens from the drug store and more recently from the dollar store. This saves me huge amounts of time and money. If I brake or lose my glasses, oh well, there goes a buck. This is how I've saved a lot of money on glasses over the years. I've moved up from 1.25 corrective lenses to 1.75 lenses on my glasses over the years. I try only to use my reading glasses when necessary. I think using glasses when not needed further deteriorates or weakens my vision.

Sometimes drug stores offer 2 for 1 sales on their glasses. This is a good way to save money and stock up on reading glasses. One time I wanted to buy a pair of glasses, but I just wanted one pair. Another guy was looking at glasses and I told him, "let's get the 2 for 1 deal". So we both got 50% off and only had to buy one pair each. Drug store glasses are better than dollar store glasses, in my opinion. I just find a pair that fits with the right corrective lenses and I'm done.

I usually carry a magnifying glass in my pocket so I don't have to bring glasses with me as much. Being a guy and having glasses almost insures me of breaking them unless I wear them constantly. Since I only need my glasses for reading, I use a magnifying glass when I'm not reading a lot. You should check with your doctor to see if a magnifying glass or drug store/cheater glasses are right for you.

As for people with nearsightedness or who need bifocals, you need to save in other ways. Your choices for vision correction aids are contacts or glasses (or perhaps corrective surgery). I guess farsighted people might also want contacts, so this is for those folks too. You should check prices before going to an eye doctor for glasses and prescriptions. Usually the larger eye glass store chains around the country or stores in a discount department store or warehouse clubs, will have the best prices for eye exams and glasses. You can also get a prescription and then get your glasses and contacts through a cheap on-line store.

While at the eye doctor, negotiate. If you have a coupon or ad from a competitor, ask the doctor if they'll match it. But more than likely, on-line prices will be cheaper than most any store. Especially if you get another set of the same glasses. If you lose or brake your glasses, you might have to go through the whole process again. Buying 2 or more pairs of the same glasses might be what you need.

To save money, don't get all the extras on your glasses. If they have all kinds of special coatings and upgrades, you probably don't need all those add-ons and the unnecessary prices that go with them.

Cheap on-line glass and contact stores are: Discountglasses, Discountcontactlenses, GlassesUSA and 1800contacts. They might have the deals that you are looking for. There are many other on-line corrective vision stores, make sure you don't use a fly by night company. I think buying contacts on-line might be a good idea. Buying glasses, with rims might not be so good. I also don't buy shoes on-line since they probably won't fit right.

If you have frames that you like, just ask the eye store to swap out your old lenses with your new ones. This can save you money and keep you from having to pick out a new style of frames.

Whenever you go to a medical provider for medical purposes, use your FSA or HSA so you'll be paying with pre-tax dollars.

If you have been wearing glasses and notice other problems with your vision or eyes, you should consult your doctor or eye doctor. The things I've done in this chapter are what I do. Consult your doctor or eye doctor about any medical problems and medical decisions.

7

How You Can Save On Prescriptions

Once again, prevention is the best medicine. If most people were to be at or get to their correct weight, they probably wouldn't need many or any prescriptions. Regular exercising and a proper diet should keep you at your weight goals. My book "How I lost 46 Lbs. In 96 Days" shows how I did it. My book also talks about the natural supplements I took, and currently take, to help me keep my high blood pressure (hawthorn berry supplement) and my type 2 diabetes (cinnamon supplement) under control.

Supplements can be used to help with people's medical conditions. There's a book by Shane Ellison M.S., "Over The Counter Natural Cures" that has loads of supplement information that can help with chronic medical conditions. Shane is a chemist. The book has recommendations for supplements to take for type 2 diabetes, high blood pressure, high cholesterol and many other ailments. These are natural ways to help chronic conditions that are also cheap. I got the idea to use supplements to help me with my conditions after reading Shane's book. The supplements I've used from his book seem to work for me. If you don't have insurance or have outrageous prescription costs, think about reading Shane's book. Even if you have good medical insurance, you should read Shane's book. You should consult your doctor and pharmacist about taking any supplements, especially if you are already taking other medications.

Ask your local pharmacist if they have something to take care for your medical problem, even before you go to the doctor.

They might give you an over the counter medicine that will take care of your health problem. Pharmacists are actually Doctors of Pharmacy. They will refer you to your doctor if needed. Before you start any workout regiment, consult your doctor. Before you take any supplements, especially if you're already on medications, consult your doctor.

There is a new primary care way of doctoring out there. It is called Direct Primary Care. I like to think of it as co-op doctors. For a low monthly fee, they will provide you and/or your family with primary care. This usually includes a yearly physical and might also include at cost or slightly above cost prescription drugs. Direct Primary Care usually doesn't take health insurance or Medicare or Medicaid. It is a new program that gets the government and insurance companies mostly out of health care. This might be a good way to go for people that have heavy prescription bills every month, especially if they don't have insurance at all. You can find a list of Direct Primary Care doctors at mapper.dpcfrontier.com. There are currently over 1150 Direct Primary Care offices throughout 48 states in the U.S. Go to a DPC's website near you to see all the benefits they offer by joining and their prices. I will talk more about DPC care in chapter 10.

If you have a chronic disease, you should find out which pharmacy has the best prices for your prescriptions. Then stick to using them. If the prices of your prescriptions start to rise, then look around again for better prices. You should always be looking around, even if you have a decent price.

Many Americans take prescription drugs. If you have or don't have insurance, then the cheapest routes for prescriptions are probably the big discount stores and warehouse clubs. One discount store currently has a special of $4 for a 30 day supply or $10 for a 90 day supply on certain generic prescription drugs. Using generic brands for prescriptions, when possible, can save you a lot.

When a doctor prescribes you medicine, ask if he could prescribe you a cheaper generic or non-generic substitute if possible. Many national pharmacies offer generic discounts on prescriptions.

On-line pharmacies might save you money, especially with 90 day supplies. Express Scripts and Healthwarehouse.com might give you a break on prices.

If you live close to the border, you may be able to buy your prescriptions in Mexico for reduced prices. Check to see if it is legal to bring your specific drugs/prescriptions across the border. Also you will need to show a prescription for the exact drugs and supply that you are bringing into the country. The FDA and Border Patrol both regulate drugs entering the U.S. You should check with both to make sure you are in compliance with U.S. laws. If you are flying, the TSA also has regulations that need to be checked. You'll also need a passport to get across the border and back.

If you don't have insurance, you should get a discount prescription card. There are many like: InsideRx, GoodRx, WeRx.org, and WellRx. These websites might also help you search for the best prices for your prescriptions and might allow you to print coupons or use their discount cards to take advantage of lower store prices. BlinkHealth displays pre-negotiated prices on their website. You pay on-line and they'll ship it to you or you can pick it up at a local pharmacy. It is best to check all these sites to maximize savings. Even if you have insurance, you should try use these programs. Some pharmacies also offer their own prescription savings club cards. Check with the pharmacy you frequent (and other stores) about their prescription programs.

There are also prescription assistance programs. If you don't have insurance or drug coverage, you might be eligible for discounted or free medications like insulin. The non-profit NeedyMeds might be able to help you find cheap or free drugs if you qualify. NeedyMeds also might provide cheap or free dental and access to medical clinics for those who qualify.

Sometimes buying your prescriptions in longer supplies (like 90 days rather than 30), can save you money. You can also visit the drug manufacturers website to see if they have saving offers or coupons.

Ask your doctor what might be the best, cheapest drug for your condition. For example, long lasting drugs, may not really be needed and might cost more. Many insurers have apps that can tell you if there is a lower cost option available. You can look it up as you talk with your doctor. Check to see if your insurance company has an app like this.

Sometimes your insurance isn't as cheap as what the stores automatically sell drugs for without insurance. One time I went into a discount store and they had generic prescriptions priced low, they said it would be cheaper without my insurance. I said "try it with my insurance any way". I saved an extra $4 dollars. So your insurance may or may not help you get the best price with their special store discounts.

If your doctor recommends you take 50 mg of a drug a day. See if your doctor can prescribe a 100 mg pill that you can split in half. They call this drug/pill splitting. The cost for a 100 mg pill probably isn't going to be much greater than a 50 mg pill. You could save a lot, especially if the drug is outrageously priced to begin with.

Always consult your doctor about taking any supplements or vitamins.

8

How You Can Save On Colonoscopies

A couple of years ago I had a colonoscopy. They say you should have it done when you hit 50. I put it off until I was 53. Then a guy I know died from colon cancer at age 52. I went and got a colonoscopy right away. Now this is supposedly preventive care. I had a good insurance program/policy but the procedure wasn't preventive care priced. The procedure cost about $9,000! That's what the bill said. I think the insurance company actually paid less, but who knows. My deductible portion was over $1000 out of my own pocket. This is ridiculous. I know people who haven't gotten a colonoscopy because of the outrageous cost and/or it's deductible. What's even worse is that the whole procedure took about 20 minutes. That means I was charged about $27,000 an hour! I must say, other than the outrageous price, I would give the hospital an A rating for everything else. I thought that because I had polyps removed, that this might be the reason it cost me so much. But I've had people tell me they had to pay high deductibles even though their test didn't find any polyps.

You should check your health insurance to see what they'll pay for and the deductible they charge for colonoscopies. You don't want a surprise huge bill. Find out where you will get your colonoscopy done, then get a referral from your primary doctor to go to them.

Imagine if you didn't have insurance. You don't get a colonoscopy because of the cost and then later you get cancer and the cost to treat you is horrendous. Worse, you get cancer and die. I checked my states' department of insurance to find out if my insurance company could charge me that much for a preventive care deductible. Yes, they said, they could. So I had to pay up. I shopped around before hand, but everyone in my area wanted about the same outrageous amount. I had one hospital not even return my e-mail for a price quote on a colonoscopy. I guess that was beneath them. It seems that pretty much everyone charges the same monopolistic prices for colonoscopies in my area. But I did find a website that might help people with or without insurance.

The website is at colonoscopyassist.com. You can go to their site and type in your city or zip code. It will show you locations that can give you screenings for cancer. The prices start at around $1100 and up for colonoscopies. They also offer other screening options for less. If you don't have insurance or have high deductible insurance or just don't want to be a party to the rip off conspiracy of colonoscopies, then you should try this website. But you should get some type of screening for colon cancer when you hit 50, or sooner if you have a family history of it. During my colonoscopy the doctor removed 6 polyps. I guess you can't get colon cancer unless you first have polyps (that's my understanding), then the polyps can go to a precancerous stage. Then they can go to a cancerous stage. So I want to get rid of any polyps before something bad happens. I'm not a doctor, check with your doctor about all the colonoscopy specifics and screenings.

Shane Ellison M.S., has a book "Over The Counter Natural Cures" that has a chapter on turmeric and its active ingredient, curcumin. This supplement apparently helps cells self destruct. My cells are programmed to die or self destruct if they get old, weak or damaged. The older I get the more likely my cells won't automatically self destruct. Curcumin apparently helps cells to self destruct when they're supposed to. Remember, Shane is a chemist. Everything in his book that I have tried, has worked for me. I take his recommended curcumin brand daily. Once again, I do not get paid to endorse any company, person, or product in this book (other than my books). Consult your doctor about any supplements you plan on taking.

9

How You Can Save If You Don't Have Health Insurance

If you have insurance or not, prevention is the best medicine. If you stop smoking, workout, eat your vegetables, drink plenty of liquids, sleep 8 hours a night and stay at your correct weight, you'll probably not be needing to see a doctor or go to the hospital much. Also, try to avoid stress. When you are stressed out, it lowers your immune system.

If you are unfortunate enough to not have

health insurance, this is bad. Not having coverage can be scary. If something bad happens it can wipe you out financially. There are many ways you can still have some relief from the stress of no coverage. When you're young, it doesn't seem as necessary to have coverage. But it's good to have some kind of health insurance regardless of your age. If you don't have insurance or don't want to spend outrageous money for health insurance, this is the chapter you need to read.

If you don't have insurance you should check to see if you are eligible for free Medicaid. You need to be low income. If you are low income you might also be eligible for your states public access health care system, if they have one. They might be the same program. You should check with your state's health care website to see if you qualify for these 2 programs. Search "Medicaid" and then your state on the internet. Search "public health access" and then your state.

If you are 65 years old, then get enrolled in Medicare. Go to medicare.gov. If you are a veteran, go to va.gov to see if you are eligible to get free or reduced cost treatment.

You can go to healthcare.gov to find if you can get low cost health insurance. This is the government's on-line health insurance comparison and shopping site. They offer insurance on a sliding scale so this might definitely help you find cheap insurance if you don't make much money.

Many times counties have hospitals (county hospitals) that are set up to help the indigent. You can call or go on-line to your county health offices' website to see what programs they have for low income people or if they have a county hospital. Search "county hospital" or "social services" or "community clinics" and then your county and state. They might also provide dental and vision care. You might need to be low income to qualify.

There are other organizations that might help with free or discounted health care. Try these websites to see if they might help you: freeclinics.com or findahealthcenter.hrsa.gov.

If you don't think you can qualify for these programs, see if your employer offers health insurance through your job. Sometimes they offer free or discounted health care for their employees and maybe their families. Sometimes employers offer just major medical/high deductible insurance to their employees at a discounted rate. Any kind of health insurance is usually good to have in case of an accident or illness.

There are walk-in clinics, that charge reasonable rates, that might see you for a flat fee. Search on-line for "walk-in clinics" and "urgent care clinics" and then your city/state. Many discount stores and pharmacies are starting to have clinics in their stores. This is a great idea. For a small fee, usually for about the price of a regular insurance co-pay, you can see a doctor or nurse practitioner. I hope this is the wave of the future (along with DPC's). When you go shopping, see if your retailer or pharmacy offers these services. You might also ask the pharmacist in these stores about these programs.

If you have a medical problem, before you

go to the doctor, go to or call your local pharmacist. If you have a skin problem, stomach ailment or other health concern, the pharmacist might give you an over the counter product. This can save on a doctor visit and perhaps expensive medications.

If you have chronic illnesses, there is a book by Shane Ellison M.S., "Over The Counter Natural Cures" that has information on natural supplements for high blood pressure, high cholesterol, diabetes, depression and many other afflictions. Shane is a chemist. This book rocks. If you don't have insurance and/or can't afford your medications, read this book. Be sure to consult a doctor or pharmacist about taking supplements, especially if you're already on medications.

I take glucosamine and boswellia supplements for my knee pains and because of them, I very seldom have pain anymore. Be sure to talk to your doctor or pharmacist about taking any supplements, especially if you're already on medications.

If you're having a baby, consider having a

midwife help with the delivery. They are trained specifically for child birthing. They run about $2000 and they know what they are doing. Chapter 15 covers this in more detail.

I've had people tell me they pay around $700 for their annual physical blood work, with insurance. Instead of paying outrageous prices for lab work for your physical (or if you don't have any insurance), go to a local lab and have them do it for cheap. Ask your provider what blood test they want you to do (generally the test will be a metabolic or chemistry test). Then make an appointment with a lab to get a blood draw for that test. Then have your doctor or one of the doctors at the lab tell you what the results mean. You could also go to an urgent care or walk-in clinic or pharmacy clinic to have their doctor or nurse practitioner explain the results to you. You can find labs on-line by searching "lab tests" or "medical tests" and your city/state. There has been an upsurge of cheap labs available to the general public that test for most everything.

Paying for your medical procedures in advance might get you discounts from the doctor and hospital.

You can go to ehealth, getinsured.com and GoHealth to find health insurance programs. You might only want to get low priced health insurance programs/policies such as major medical. This will cover the serious situations, but not runny noses. If you had a major medical insurance policy and just went to walk-in clinics for the little things, you might have most of your health care concerns covered. Figure out the health insurance plan that is best for your needs.

On your homeowners policy, you could increase your medical payouts per person and per incident, in case you're hurt at home. You might also increase your car insurance policy for medical payouts in case you're in a major accident. Both these 2 adjustments to your policies probably won't cost you a lot extra and you'd be somewhat covered at home or in your car (and also other people) for many serious accidents and medical expenses. Talk to your insurance agent about these additional coverages. Your work probably covers you for on the job injuries.

Another option to use with high deductible/major medical insurance is the Direct Primary Care clinics that are becoming popular. They generally don't except insurance. I'll talk more about them in the next chapter.

If you don't have dental or health insurance, you might try medical tourism. I talk more about this in chapter 16. Even if you have insurance, medical tourism might be the way to go for some medical and dental procedures.

This chapter is specifically for people that don't have insurance and would have no regular access to a doctor's advice. It is best to consult a doctor about any health care problems. Consult your insurance agent about health insurance and home owners insurance policies and there ramifications.

10

How You Can Save With Direct Primary Care Clinics

Direct Primary Care (DPC) clinics are popping up everywhere. These clinics are usually owned by the doctor(s) and they take patients in as members. The monthly fees are usually anywhere from $50-$100 a month for a single person, they also usually offer low cost family plans. Each practice charges their own different fees. They also offer different services for their fee. This is like a gym membership or a membership to a wholesale club. DPC's take care of your basic primary care, not most surgeries. Check with each Direct Primary Care to see what services they offer.

Many of these clinics offer unlimited communications with the doctor, either in person, by e-mail, by phone or by on-line video. The clinics may also offer yearly physicals. They also might offer discounted blood work, prescriptions and x-rays. There are currently over 1150 DPC clinics throughout the continual 48 states.

You can find a DPC clinic near you at dpc.frontier.com. This site shows the locations of the clinics and how you can contact them and/or their websites. The good thing about DPC's are that they promote wellness rather than sickness. When I had a weight problem my doctor constantly tried to get me on medications for diabetes and high blood pressure. Never did he mention to me that I should exercise and loose weight to correct my medical issues. Not once.

Since the DPC doctor has everything to gain (time and less stress) by keeping you healthy, he will be   prescribing prevention.

The DPC doctor is innately geared towards prevention. My regular doctor must have felt, the more times I see this guy, the more money I can make. This is sad if you think about it. Many DPC's don't take Medicare, Medicaid or health insurance.

It would be best if you do decide to join a Direct Primary Care clinic (I think of them as co-op doctors) to also have a major medical/catastrophic/high deductible insurance policy in place in case something major happens. With high deductible health insurance you can also get a HSA. If the government would give people vouchers to pay for DPC clinics rather than Medicare and Medicaid insurance (in conjunction with major medical insurance), then we'd probably fix skyrocketing costs overnight. I think Direct Primary Care is the best route for America's health care. To promote health care, rather than sick care, can only be good for America.

11

How You Can Save With Micro Hospitals

Micro hospitals are also popping up around the country. These mini hospitals generally provide about 80% to 90% of the services that a larger hospital can provide. They are many times owned by the doctors who work there. These hospitals generally charge less and provide faster services than regular hospitals. Micro hospitals are usually priced above an average urgent care clinic, but generally far less than regular hospitals.

They can also help make hospitals

available in smaller rural areas, that generally wouldn't be able to support a larger hospital. A lot of these new hospitals are built in areas that have a shortage of regular hospital beds and services. Micro hospitals generally have emergency, pharmacy, lab and imagery departments. They also have less rooms because they usually only have patients in their hospital for up to 48 hours. Patients needing longer hospital stays are generally transferred to other facilities.

Many corporations are having their employees go to these micro hospitals to save employer costs. The micro hospitals average 8 to 10 beds per hospital. They are open 24/7 and year round. The hospitals are usually tailored to the need of the specific community they are in. Most micro hospitals are not level one trauma centers and they end up transferring about 5% of their patients to larger hospitals with more services.

The costs of micro hospitals are generally lower. Some of these hospitals don't take Medicare or Medicaid so they don't have all the extra red tape. Since the costs of these hospitals tend to be less, this would probably make your deductibles also less. You should check with your insurer to see if the micro hospital you plan on going to is in their provider network or you could have huge bills later. But if you don't have insurance, this might be a cheaper avenue than regular hospitals in emergencies and for many medical operations and procedures.

You can find these hospitals on the internet by searching for "mini hospitals" or "micro hospitals" or "neighborhood hospitals" and then your city and state.

12

How You Can Get Affordable Health Insurance

If you don't have health insurance than the best way to keep from having high medical bills is prevention. You should get to your correct weight, exercise, eat a healthy diet, don't smoke, drink in moderation or not at all. These are the habits that will help keep you away from the doctor.

Hopefully your employer offers health insurance but if they don't, there are options. The trick is to find the best and cheapest coverage for your particular needs. You'll need to decide if you want premium or lesser health insurance coverage, especially after reading about Direct Primary Care clinics in chapter 10. Sometimes people might only have a small amount of money that can go towards their health care every month and they want as much protection as they can afford.

You should consider not just the things the policy covers and the premium, but also the deductible. If you are young and healthy, you might just want a higher deductible health insurance policy because there is a good chance you won't need to go to a doctor or hospital. Usually the higher the premium, the less the deductible and vice versa.

If you qualify for VA benefits, you might be able to get low cost or free medical care through them. Go to va.gov to find out more. If you are low income you may qualify for free medical care through medicaid.gov. Go to their site to find out more. If you are 65 years old or disabled, you may qualify for Medicare. Go to their website at medicare.gov to find out more.

The government set up a website that you can go to at healthcare.gov that allows you to search for and purchase premium health insurance programs. You fill out your information and then you'll be given options for insurance that you can enroll for. These programs usually have a lot of coverage and are considered premium programs. Your costs will be on a sliding basis, if you make less, you pay less. This might be a good place to start your insurance search, especially if you don't make much money.

Currently to buy health insurance, the insurance company needs to be authorized to sell in your state. There has been moves to make all insurance companies able to sell nationally, this is a good idea for more competition. Obviously in the smaller populated states, there will be less insurance companies wanting to sell there. This could lead to monopolistic tendencies when there is limited competition and would probably lead to higher premiums and deductibles.

If you are shopping for low priced health

insurance or any insurance, it is usually best to go to an insurance broker. A broker is an agent that sells multiple company's policies and they can shop around for you. Brokers will be able to find all kinds of insurance programs, not just premium programs. They can also shop for major medical, catastrophic and high deductible policies. This might be a good way to go to save some cash, if you feel you don't need all the bells and whistles of premium insurance or if you plan on joining a Direct Primary Care clinic. Search the internet for "health insurance broker" and then your state or by your city/state.

On-line insurance websites like ehealth, getinsured.com and gohealth would also be a good places to shop. These should have broker like searches for health insurance policies.

You can go to a specific insurance companies website, but you'll only get their rates. But you could possibly find a sweet deal only offered on-line, so if you have time you might consider that. Your state department of insurance has a list of insurance companies authorized to sell health insurance in your state. Call your state's department of insurance or go to their website to get a list of these health insurance companies. Search "department of insurance" and your state.

If you work for someone as an independent contractor or if you are self employed, you may be able to get insurance through your group, organization or association that covers everyone in your field of employment. An example might be if you are a plumber and belong to a plumber's union or association, they might offer group insurance. This might be a good way to save, since there might be discounted rates. If you belong to an association in your field or business, call up their headquarters or go to their website on-line to see if they have group health insurance that can save you money.

There are also health sharing plans that offer health coverage. Medishare.com, Liberty Health Share and other Christian groups offer coverage that might save you money. This is not technically insurance. Everyone in the group pays into the program each month in premiums and then the non-profit pays out the bills. These programs might have guidelines for participating. You can ask your minister or priest or rabbi or other church elder/leader if your congregation has a program that they already subscribe to. You'll want to check with your medical provider to see if they accept your share plan before joining.

Make sure any health provider you go to will take your insurance before you go to them. If you are checking your network providers, you shouldn't have to worry.

Always check with your doctor about any medical concerns. Consult with your health insurance agent about the insurance policy that would be best for you and your family.

13

How You Can Save If You Have Health Insurance

If you have regular health insurance, that covers most everything, then there are ways to save. First, prevention is the best medicine. Even if you have the best health insurance on the planet, staying healthy is cheaper. Try to be at your correct weight, this will help keep you away from the doctors, hospitals and pharmacists. Read my book "How I Lost 46 lbs. In 96 days" to see the things I did to lose my weight. If we don't lose weight America, our health care costs will always be much higher than they could be.

Get a physical, with blood work, every year. When you have a physical make sure they do a prostate check with a finger, not just a PSA test. Also get a colonoscopy and other preventive screenings when they are recommended. Get your mammograms done when suggested. Use the buddy system to give breast checks before and between recommended mammograms. Catching a medical problem early can not only save you money, but could save your life. Check your health insurance policy to see what preventive care they cover. In chapter 17 I'll discuss ways to save on mammograms.

Make sure that any referrals your doctor makes is to an in-network provider. If he sends you to his orthopedic surgeon friend, and he's not in your insurance providers network, this will probably end up costing you a lot. Always get a referral from your doctor for any procedure you get. This tells the insurance company that your doctor ordered it.

If your doctor wants you to get an MRI, check and see how much your imagery charges will be for where he wants you to go. If the amount is more than a $1000, you should shop around. Call up local stand alone imagery clinics in your area and see what they charge for the same image. Call up local urgent care clinics and see what they charge. Make sure they are in-network first. If they have much better rates, make an appointment with them. Get a referral to them from your doctor. Make sure it is the exact same imagery shot/picture though. You will probably be paying a deductible for the MRI. If this is 10%, and you find a MRI that saves you $2000, then you just saved yourself $200. Not bad for a few phone calls. You can also search "MRI" and your city/state on-line to find imagery locations.

Make sure before you have any major surgery done, that your insurance is going to cover it. Check to see if the provider performing the operation or procedure is in-network. If not, find alternatives before you might owe $10,000 out of pocket.

Make sure your health insurance covers

only the health care items you need or want. Premium insurance usually costs way more than simple major medical insurance. Also, usually by having a higher deductible, you'll usually get a lower monthly premium and vice versa. If you are young or healthy you might want to consider a higher deductible.

A great way to save on taxes is to use a Flexible Savings Account, Health Savings Account or Health Reimbursement account. These 3 programs allow you to use pre-tax dollars to pay for your medical expenses. These 3 programs have tax implications. You should talk with your tax attorney or CPA about these matters, especially if you're self employed. If you are employed, and your employer provides these different pre-tax health savings plan options, you should talk with your human resources department about them. There are whole books written about this subject. But you should get one of these to save money, especially if you usually have high health care expenses.

If you have health insurance, the most important thing to consider is your in-network care providers. Most regular insurance companies have providers that are contracted through your insurance provider for set prices. If you use those providers, then the insurance company will usually pay 100% (minus your deductible and co-pay) of the charges.

If you go to an out of network provider, your insurer might only pay 0-70% of the cost. You will be responsible for the balance. It is direly important that you find out who your in-network providers are through your insurance company. Write down the names, addresses and phone numbers of these hospitals, clinics and walk-in clinics (or print out a list of them). Do not go to any provider unless they are on that list. Obviously if it is an emergency and you're on vacation, use your judgment. Perhaps call your insurance company to get advice before you go.

Many health insurance plans have maximum deductibles for the year. You might only have to pay a $1000 towards your deductible, and your employer or insurance company with provide the rest. If you plan on getting surgeries, get them all done in the same health insurance calender year to avoid paying the maximum deductible again next year. If it is near the end of the year and you haven't had any surgeries, put off the surgery until next year (if you can). If you have a family plan, get everyone's surgeries done in one calendar year.

If you have premium insurance then maybe just having a doctor deliver your baby would be cheaper and easier. But if you have high deductible insurance or no insurance, instead of going to the hospital and having a doctor help give birth, think about trying a midwife. Their fees are usually around $2000. Midwifes have been delivering babies for 100's of years. Chapter 15 has more information on this subject.

Review your bills immediately and contact the office manager or billing/coding department in the hospital or clinic that provided you service if you see any errors. Get an itemized bill. There is more on this subject in the next chapter.

If you think you have a medical problem, go to the doctor. Don't wait until it gets serious or perhaps inoperable. On the flip side, if you have a runny nose, you might not want to rush to the doctor immediately.

If you need help with your kidneys by having dialysis, then home treatment might be for you. This would save Medicare, Medicaid and insurance companies a lot of money. But what's in it for you? You won't have to go down to the hospital or clinic and spend a whole day there. You might save on deductibles. You might not miss days of work. Usually clinical dialysis is required 3 times a week. By doing home dialysis this can save you a lot of time, money and travel. The best part is that you can do your dialysis while you're sleeping so you're not out any time by doing it. Check with your doctor to see if this might be an option for you.

If your insurance doesn't cover a medical or dental procedure you want or need, or if your deductible for the procedure is sky high, then maybe medical tourism might be the solution to your problem. You can find out more in chapter 17.

Ask questions of your doctor. If he says to have surgery, ask them if it is really necessary. Maybe there are other options. Maybe by waiting a month, the problem might get better. But ask because, why not? This is especially true of tests, drugs and x-rays that really might not be needed.

If you are quoted a price for a procedure, check on-line at HealthcareBluebook.com or fairhealthconsumer.org to see what the going rates are for these procedures in your area. Use this information to negotiate. Your deductible is usually based on the cost of the procedure. Saving $5000 on an operation could put $500 in your pocket. Especially check on the prices of MRI's. If it is essential that you have the test, x-ray or operation, shop around for a good fair price.
"

When you go to a hospital, have your doctor admit you as an "impatient". Inpatient billing usually pays for most everything your insurance covers. Outpatient and observation might have you paying a lot of your own money. Check your insurance policy or with your insurance company for this before you go to the hospital, especially if you have Medicare.

Going to the walk-in clinic instead of the emergency room can save you a small fortune. Make sure that it is in-network and is attached or near a regular hospital. Then, if your condition is serious, they can easily do a major procedure on you. You need to know the locations of your in-network providers BEFORE you have an emergency.

If you go to the hospital by ambulance, have them take you to the in-network provider's hospital, unless they think they need to go to the nearest hospital.

Always speak with your doctor about any medical concern. Consult with your insurance agent about the different health insurance policies that might be best for you and your family. Go over your insurance policy to find out the policies they have concerning your medical treatments and procedures.

14

How You Can Save On Your Medical Bills

The best way to save on your medical bills is to stay at your proper weight. Prevention is the best medicine. If you eat healthy and stay slim, your need for medical help should be reduced.

When you get your bill from the doctor or provider or hospital, make sure all the charges are accurate. Get an itemized bill and go over it line by line to see that everything looks correct. Call if you have any questions about the bill or bill coding.

Dispute any discrepancies you might find as soon as possible. They may have charged you for the wrong billing code number. You may have been charged for brain surgery instead of a brain scan. Call and inquire. Don't be rude. If you can go down to their office in person it is even better. People tend to be more helpful and friendlier when you are there in person. Ask them to take off the charge or change the price of the charge. Go to Health Care Bluebook on-line or fairhealthconsumer.org before you call or see them, to see what the going rates for procedures are in your area. If your bill has a charge that is out of line, call and question it.

If you get deductible charges from your insurance company that you don't think you should have to pay, call up your insurance company and explain your concern. If they still want you to pay up, file an appeal with your insurance company. There may be time deadlines. If you don't get satisfaction from them, you can also contact your state's department of insurance and tell them about your situation. Insurance companies authorized to sell in your state are regulated by your state's department of insurance.

My dad had a claims issue with a hospital. He didn't have insurance. They wanted something like $10,000 for an emergency room procedure. I told him to call down to billing and tell them that you don't have the money (which he didn't). Tell them you can give them what you have. They ended up taking just a couple thousand. It is better for them to get something than nothing. When hospitals sell their bad debt to collection companies, they usually just get about 10% of the owed amount. So if the hospital knows I'm not going to be able to pay them, then they might be happy with the 10% or more from me than from the collection agency. Hospitals bill on a billing sheet called "chargemaster rates". This is what a walk-in person, with no insurance pays. Insurance companies usually don't pay these outrageous charges. Why should you?

My three rules to negotiating are: never make the first offer, never accept the first offer and don't be afraid to walk away from the deal (the person who wants the deal the most, loses).

If you can make payments to the hospital or doctor, this is better than bad credit. Bad credit will blemish your credit report for usually 7 years.

If you don't feel you are tough enough to go up against the office manager or the hospital billing department, you might consider getting the help of a health advocate. This is a person who negotiates on your behalf. The company you work for may provide this service. You can also find them on-line by searching "health advocate" or "medical bill negotiators" and then your city and/or state. If you can't afford to hire one, the Patients Advocate Foundation might handle your case for free. Look them up on-line and contact them. You could also call a lawyer, sometimes just a call from an attorney can clear things up.

Keep all your bills and medical records in case a problem over billing arises. Get an itemized statement of your bill. Check for errors.

When paying your insurance bill ask if they will give you a "paid in full" discount for people who pay all at once in a timely fashion. This could get you an instant savings of 10-30%. Do the same for any outstanding hospital or provider bills.

You get a bill from the hospital or clinic after the insurance company has paid everything, but they still want more money. Make sure your insurance company has paid everything that it was supposed to pay. If it is correct, then call the provider, hospital, clinic or doctor and tell them your insurance didn't pay the whole bill and you still owe money, but you weren't anticipating this large bill. Ask how they can help you with this? Then wait and see what they say.

After you've tried the above techniques, ask the hospital or clinic (or insurance company) if there are any other discounts that might apply to you.

Ask the hospital or clinic if they have any Charity Care Programs that might help with your bill. Some hospitals have this for low income people.

After you've negotiated with the hospital

or provider for all you can, then ask if you could get an interest free loan to pay for the rest of the balance. Providers generally will allow 2 years to repay the balance.

Finally, the number one reason for bankruptcies in the US is medical issues. Bankruptcies are often the only solution. For example, if you owe $100,000 on medical bills and no one will work with you, don't be afraid to pick up the phone and talk to a bankruptcy attorney. Remember, in a normal world that $100,000 of medical debt would probably only been around $10,000 or $20,000. If you don't believe you'll be able to pay the hospital or provider what they say you owe them, call an attorney and get their advice.

Regardless of everything I've mentioned in this chapter, I'm not a lawyer and I'm not giving legal advice. You should consult a lawyer about any legal or tax matter or questions.

15

How You Can Save Money When Having A Baby

No medical insurance? High deductible? Maybe a midwife might work for you. A midwife is a trained medical person that specializes in the delivery of babies. The average cost of a midwife's services is around $2000. This could be less than your insurance deductible for using a regular doctor. A friend of mine had all 4 of his children delivered with the help of a midwife. If you plan on a natural child birth, then this might be the route for you.

Midwives might also have payment plans and a sliding scale for low income people. Midwives have been helping with child births for 100's of years.

In 1998 about 2.5% of the population used a midwife for child birth. By 2008 the number had risen to 7.5%. Midwives only perform regular child births. You can search for midwives at birthcenters.org or midwife.org. You should also search "midwife" and your city and state. I've noticed since midwives have became popular again, hospitals are trying to get in on the action. Try to find a midwife that isn't employed by a hospital, this will save you the cost of the middleman. We're trying to bring down the cost of medicine, not raise it.

If your doctor thinks you have a high risk pregnancy, then you should probably have the baby delivered in or near a hospital.

Medicaid helps cover the cost of child birth for low income people that qualify. Go to medicaid.gov to see if you qualify.

County hospitals often deliver babies for

little or no costs if you are low income or don't have insurance. Check on-line for a county hospital that might provide this type of service. I know a couple of people that have had babies for practically nothing at the county hospital. Search "county hospital" or "social services" and your county and/or city and state.

If you have a baby in a regular hospital, share a hospital room and save. Also, leave the hospital as soon as possible. If you can get out in 1 day, you'll save on all the extra daily charges.

Get an itemized bill and check it over for errors, before you pay. Read chapter 14 if you find any disputable items on your bill.

Find a doctor who charges a flat rate for the whole procedure, including the hospital charges. Doctors usually are affiliated with a hospital and are usually given set flat fees.

Compare hospital costs if you have your delivery at a local hospital. This sounds cheap, but why would you want to spend a lot on having a baby?   This could save you money on your deductible.

If you can do it, you could also go to another state and have your baby. The costs of child birth through a hospital is generally anywhere from $5,000 to $12,000 in the U.S. For a C section it is generally about $7,500 to $16,000. The southern states tend to have the cheaper rates, while the northeast states have the most expensive (for the most part) rates for child birth. If you don't have insurance, this could save you $1,000's by just driving or flying a little bit, especially for C sections when you know when the baby will be born.

Check to see if the hospital offers low income help. Many hospitals offer reduced fees if you qualify for low income status.

Use your FSA or HSA account to use pre-tax dollars.

Have your delivery and other surgeries and procedures in the same calendar year to save on your deductible charges if you can.

Paying for a delivery in advance might get you savings from your doctor, hospital and/or midwife.

Skip the options. Don't have the epidural and save money. Don't have your baby circumcised and save money. Don't have photos done through the hospital, do them yourself. Ask if any procedure, drugs or service is really necessary.

Make sure your doctor and hospital are in-network. This is probably the most important question for people with insurance. Make sure your insurance also covers all the procedures you'll need. If you get an epidural and your insurance doesn't pay for it, it could cost you a $1,000 out of pocket.

Be sure to talk to your doctor about any and all medical matters and concerns.

16

How You Can Save With Medical Tourism

What is the best way to save on medical expenses? Prevention, Prevention, Prevention.

Recently there has been a rise in medical tourism. This involves leaving the good old USA to have medical procedures and surgeries done in other countries. The reason they call it tourism is because it is usually in conjunction with a trip to a pretty country. You might save anywhere from 40-85% on health care costs, and get a nice vacation. If you don't have insurance, you should definitely consider this option. Surgeries in other countries aren't cheap, its just that in the U.S. it sometimes costs many times more for the same procedures. This makes it seem like the other countries might not know what they're doing by their costs. The idea of "you get what you pay for", doesn't usually apply to American medical costs.

If you have good health insurance it might not make sense to go elsewhere. Although medical technology is great in many countries, you might want the piece of mind of staying in America. There's a book "Patients Beyond Borders" by Josef Woodman that has great information on how to correctly do medical tourism. In the book he talks about the $6,000 rule. If your procedure in the U.S. is $6,000 or more, then you can probably have in done overseas and get a free vacation for about the same price. If you live close to the Mexican border, then the $6,000 rule might be less since you won't have all the associated travel costs.

Keep in mind many of the doctors in the U.S. have been trained in India and other medically advanced countries. So the idea of having surgery in those countries isn't so crazy. Countries that have a lot of medical tourism are: Mexico, Costa Rica, Thailand and India. There are also many other countries, pretty much everywhere, that offer less cost for procedures than in the U.S. Many people go to these countries for elective surgeries (like cosmetic) or other procedures that aren't covered by their insurance policies. Americans also often go down to Mexico to get cheap dental work and dentures.

Check with your insurance company to see if they'll pay for all or part of your surgery outside of the country. If it will save them money and the procedure is on your policy, they should be very receptive. Check with them to see their requirements. Also, check to see if your insurance company might already have a medical travel package in place designed for your procedure. This might make it the best and easiest way to get a free vacation and medical procedure at minimal costs.

Why would you want to go to another

country if you have good health insurance? If it saves your insurance company $50,000, then it could save you $5,000 or more on your deductible. If you're not going to save anything because of a low deductible, then you might just stay in the U.S. If you don't have insurance or your insurance doesn't cover your procedure, or it's just cheaper for you because of a high deductible, then maybe medical tourism will work for you.

If you do go to other countries for surgery or dental work, just make sure the hospitals, clinics and labs you use are on an accredited medical list. One list is the non-profit Joint Commission International list of health care providers. This is an organization, related to the Joint Commission, that checks out medical facilities for job performance, cleanliness and etc. (about 21,000 facilities in the U.S are accredited by the Joint Commission). There are presently about 600 hospitals and clinics that are JCI approved outside of the U.S. There are other accreditation organizations that might also ease your mind. Some of them cater to certain specialties in their medical field. If you live close to the border, ask around to get recommendations on south of the border dental clinics.

You can search the JointCommisionInternational.org site for hospitals or clinics that can perform your procedure. Then check the prices and locations of the hospitals to determine which hospital you'd like to have your procedure done at. You might want to check costs of flights and hotels first to get an idea of your overall costs for that destination's procedure.

If you are serious about medical tourism, I suggest you read "Patients Beyond Borders" to find out exactly how to go about it. There are other good books about medical tourism out there as well. You might also want to consult a medical travel professional through the American Tourism Association. Patientsbeyondborders.com has a list of recommended providers on it and they also offer consultation. Trips outside of the U.S. will require passports and possibly visas. This is something you might need to plan ahead for. You also might need to get booster shots or new vaccinations.

Consult your doctor before you make plans to go on your medical tourism trip. Also, consult your insurance company concerning their requirements. You should do your research before you decide to go. I have never done medical tourism, but in 2017 over 1.4 million Americans apparently sought medical tourism.

17

How You Can Save On Mammograms

Breast cancer is responsible for the deaths of over 40,000 women each year in the U.S. The death rate has been falling greatly for the last 30 years due primarily to early detection. Prevention for breast cancer would be self examinations and mammograms.

Early detection is the key. If nothing else you should be doing a monthly breast exam. You can go to nationalbreastcancer.org and they have a page "breast self exam". This will show you the correct way to do a monthly exam. If you find something you think is wrong during your exam, go see your doctor immediately.

If you have premium health insurance, under the Affordable Care Act, you should be able to get mostly free screenings starting at age 40. If you don't have health insurance or just high deductible health insurance that doesn't cover mammograms, there are many other ways to get free or reduced cost mammograms.

The National Breast Cancer Foundation partners with facilities to give free mammograms to women that might not have other options. You can find out more at nationalbreastcancer.org.

You can also check with komen.org to find a location or affiliate that offers free mammograms in your area. You can also call them at 1-877-go-komen (1-877-465-6636).

The government also offers a program through the CDC (Center for Disease Control). This program offers free exams to qualified low income people. You can find out more at CDC.gov. You can also search "CDC" and "breast cancer screenings". The program is called The National Breast and Cervical Cancer Early Detection Program. The only draw back is that the free screenings tend to only be in a state capitals, but check anyway.

Some YWCA's also provide breast cancer screenings to qualified people. You can go to their website at ywca.org to find out more.

The American Breast Cancer Foundation also has a program designed to help low income or uninsured people get financial assistance in paying for mammograms. You can find out more at Abcf.org or search for "ABCF" and "breast cancer assistance program".

Some imagery centers offer discounted mammograms during cancer awareness month. Search for "imagery centers" and your city/state. Call them up and see if they have any specials.

If you have Medicare or Medicaid, they

should cover mammograms.

In conclusion use prevention and price comparisons to help lower our nation's health care costs. It's everyones responsibility to bring down our health care costs.

Ask your doctor any questions about your medical concerns. Talk to an attorney about any legal matters. Consult your insurance agent about any health insurance policy questions and advice.

Thanks for reading this book!

18

Other Books By Brian Orvik

Non-Fiction-

How I Lost 46 Lbs. In 96 Days

How You Can Save Up To $57,000 On College!

Fiction-

Terror Wheel: A John Smart Novel

www.ingramcontent.com/pod-product-compliance
Lightning Source LLC
Chambersburg PA
CBHW031258250726
48655CB00005B/2261